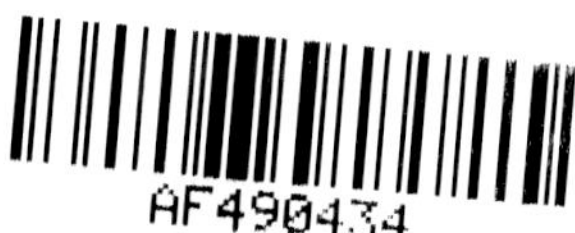

THiS JOURNAL
BELONGS TO

____

____

www.ingramcontent.com/pod-product-compliance
Lightning Source LLC
Chambersburg PA
CBHW051443150726
48000CB00005B/2228

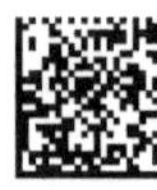

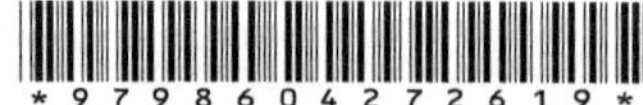